Heroes of the
COVID-19 PANDEMIC

Barbara Sheen

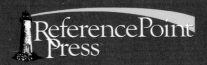

ReferencePoint
Press

San Diego, CA

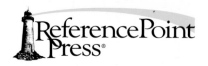

About the Author

Barbara Sheen is the author of 107 books for young people. She lives in New Mexico with her family. In her spare time she likes to swim, garden, walk, cook, and read.

© 2021 ReferencePoint Press, Inc.
Printed in the United States

For more information, contact:
ReferencePoint Press, Inc.
PO Box 27779
San Diego, CA 92198
www.ReferencePointPress.com

Picture Credits:

Cover: Sara Carpenter/Shutterstock.com
 8: Jason Whitman/Shutterstock.com
12: Pordee_Aomboon/Shutterstock.com
16: Halfpoint/Shutterstock.com
19: insta_photos/Shutterstock.com
23: Travelpixs/Shutterstock.com
26: Associated Press

31: Laurel Smith/ZUMA Press/Newscom
35: CNP/AdMedia/SIPA/Newscom
39: Kyodo/Newscom
43: Associated Press
47: Antonio Marquez Lanza/Shutterstock.com
49: Associated Press
53: Prostock-Studio/iStock

LIBRARY OF CONGRESS CATALOGING-IN-PUBLICATION DATA

Names: Sheen, Barbara, author.
Title: Heroes of the COVID-19 pandemic / by Barbara Sheen.
Description: San Diego, CA : ReferencePoint Press, Inc., 2021. | Series:
  Understanding the COVID-19 pandemic | Includes bibliographical
  references and index.
Identifiers: LCCN 2020046312 (print) | LCCN 2020046313 (ebook) | ISBN
  9781678200367 (library binding) | ISBN 9781678200374 (ebook)
Subjects: LCSH: COVID-19 Pandemic, 2020---Juvenile literature. | Disaster
  relief--History--21st century--Juvenile literature.
Classification: LCC RA653.5 .S54 2021 (print) | LCC RA653.5 (ebook) | DDC
  362.1962/414--dc23
LC record available at https://lccn.loc.gov/2020046312
LC ebook record available at https://lccn.loc.gov/2020046313

CONTENTS

The COVID-19 Pandemic:
The First Nine Months of 2020

January

(11) China reports first known death from mysterious virus that infected dozens in Wuhan in December.

(20) WHO reports that Japan, South Korea, and Thailand have first confirmed virus cases outside of mainland China.

(30) WHO declares global health emergency.

(31) US restricts travel from China.

February

(2) Philippines reports first coronavirus death outside of China.

(5) Japan quarantines *Diamond Princess* cruise ship; within 2 weeks the ship has more than 600 infections.

(11) WHO names the disease caused by the new coronavirus COVID-19 (for *coronavirus disease 2019*).

(23) Europe's first major outbreak occurs in Italy.

(26) Brazil has Latin America's first known case of coronavirus.

March

(13) US president Donald Trump officially declares national emergency.

(19) California becomes first US state to enact statewide shutdown.

(24) Officials announce 1-year postponement of 2020 Tokyo Summer Olympics.

(26) US becomes world leader in confirmed coronavirus infections.

(27) President Trump signs $2 trillion economic stimulus bill sent to him by Congress.

April

(2) Pandemic shutdowns have cost nearly 10 million Americans their jobs.

(10) Coronavirus cases surge in Russia.

(14) IMF warns of worst global downturn since Great Depression.

(17) President Trump encourages protests of social distancing restrictions.

(26) Pandemic has killed more than 200,000 and sickened more than 2.8 million worldwide.

(30) Several major airlines begin requiring face masks.

May

1 FDA authorizes remdesivir as an emergency treatment for COVID-19.

17 Japan and Germany fall into recession.

26 Widespread protests begin after George Floyd is killed by Minneapolis police; because many protesters wear masks, feared virus outbreaks do not occur.

27 US has more than 100,000 COVID-19 deaths, surpassing all other nations.

June

4 Previously spared regions of Middle East, Latin America, Africa, and South Asia have large spikes.

11 Coronavirus cases in Africa exceed 200,000, with one-fourth in South Africa.

20 Florida and South Carolina are among 19 US states experiencing sharp rise in new infections.

28 Final phase of clinical trials for AstraZeneca–University of Oxford COVID-19 vaccine begins in Brazil.

July

11 For the first time, President Trump wears a mask during a public appearance.

16 Georgia's governor rescinds local government mask mandates.

17 After easing restrictions in May, skyrocketing infections force India to reimpose lockdown.

27 Final phase of clinical trials for Moderna COVID-19 vaccine begins in the US.

August

9 New Zealand achieves 100 days without a new diagnosis of coronavirus.

11 Amid global skepticism, Russia announces first approved-for-use coronavirus vaccine.

17 Democrats begin first-ever, all-virtual convention to nominate the party's presidential candidate, Joe Biden.

23 FDA authorizes convalescent plasma as an emergency treatment for COVID-19.

27 Before a crowd of about 1,500 people, President Trump accepts Republican presidential nomination.

September

8 Nine of the leading drug companies developing COVID-19 vaccines pledge in writing to put safety before speed.

21 President Trump tells supporters at an Ohio rally that COVID "affects virtually nobody."

30 The pandemic has killed more than 1 million people and sickened nearly 34 million worldwide. In the US, the pandemic has killed nearly 207,000 people and sickened more than 7 million. Two days later, on October 2, President Trump tweets that he and First Lady Melania Trump have tested positive for the virus that causes COVID-19.

Based on Derrick Bryson Taylor, "A Timeline of the Coronavirus Pandemic," *New York Times*, July 21, 2020. www.nytimes.com.

Ordinary People Doing Extraordinary Things

Navjot Arora is a Westchester County, New York, restaurant owner. In the early months of the COVID-19 pandemic, his restaurant was shuttered, as were thousands of other businesses all over the world. Millions of people lost their jobs, including approximately one in four US restaurant workers, according to the Independent Restaurant Coalition. Without a steady income, many of these individuals could not afford to buy food. Arora wanted to help feed food-insecure restaurant and hospitality workers in his area. In March 2020 he and fellow restaurant owners in his community vowed to make 1 million gallons (3.8 million L) of soup, which they planned to offer to people in need. When local businesses heard about the project, they donated food and money to the group, which also set up a GoFundMe page. By July 2020 the soup makers had made and distributed soup to thousands of people. As Arora explains, "We're all in this together. . . . The only thing we can all do is try to help. For me that means feeding people. . . . You can either be paralyzed in fear or you can decide to do something. I'm making soup."[1]

A Devastating Pandemic

Arora was not alone in his actions. Many people have stepped up to help others during the COVID-19 pandemic. A pandemic is a disease outbreak that spreads over large geographic areas, such as whole countries, continents, or multiple countries and continents, and affects a large portion of the population.

In December 2019 a new virus—part of a family of coronaviruses that cause everything from the common cold to the respiratory illness known as SARS—arose in China. It causes a serious illness known as COVID-19 (for *coronavirus disease 2019*).

> "You can either be paralyzed in fear or you can decide to do something."[1]
>
> —Navjot Arora, chef and restaurant owner

The virus spread like wildfire, triggering a worldwide pandemic. As it raced around the globe, it impacted the lives of almost every person and society, leaving illness, death, and economic hardship in its wake. In an attempt to slow the spread of the disease, cities, states, and entire countries locked down. Businesses, schools, places of worship, and other public venues closed. People socially isolated themselves, sheltering in place in their homes. Still, the virus managed to devastate society. According to the World Health Organization, as of October 6, 2020, there were more than 35 million confirmed cases of COVID-19 and over 1 million deaths worldwide. By that date, the United States alone reported more than 7 million cases and more than 213,000 deaths. In addition, millions of people became unemployed, leading to the largest global economic recession in modern history.

Going Above and Beyond

Throughout the crisis, people of diverse ages and backgrounds have put the needs of others above their own, often at great personal sacrifice. They have performed acts of service and kindness

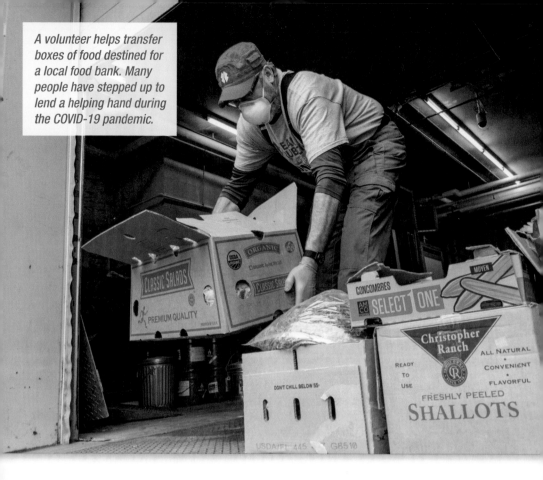

A volunteer helps transfer boxes of food destined for a local food bank. Many people have stepped up to lend a helping hand during the COVID-19 pandemic.

to help and support sick and vulnerable people, keep society safe and functioning, contain and control the virus, and help their local communities. Many of these individuals are health care professionals, first responders, and other frontline and essential workers. Others include but are not limited to scientists, public health professionals, and young volunteers. For instance, Whitney, a young medical technologist who works in a Virginia hospital, has risked being exposed to the virus on a daily basis. As part of her job, she analyzes hundreds of potentially infectious COVID-19 test swabs. Because of the overwhelming number of samples sent to her laboratory and the importance of getting test results back quickly, she has often worked late into the night. Even though doing her job has endangered her health, Whitney has not quit. She, like thousands of other selfless individuals, has put the needs of others above her own.

What Makes a Hero?

Because of their unselfish acts, many of these individuals have been called heroes. Social scientists do not have a single definition of what constitutes a hero, but almost all agree that heroes are individuals who perform selfless acts in the service of others. Often, these actions involve personal risk or sacrifice. In addition, studies suggest that heroes share certain personality traits, such as empathy, selflessness, determination, and the ability to face fear. Despite exhibiting these traits and performing heroic actions, many of the people who have been dubbed heroes during the COVID-19 pandemic do not consider themselves heroes. They insist that they are average people who care about and want to help others, either by doing the jobs they trained for or through small and large acts of kindness. As Sharon O'Neill, a nurse practitioner and the vice chair of the University of Southern California's Department of Nursing, contends, "When you're in the middle of dealing with something like this . . . you don't think of yourself as a hero. You think of it as your job, what you've signed up for. It's a privilege to take care of these people."[2] Indeed, no matter what they are called, in response to the COVID-19 pandemic, many ordinary people have done extraordinary things.

> "When you're in the middle of dealing with something like this . . . you don't think of yourself as a hero. You think of it as your job, what you've signed up for."[2]
>
> —Sharon O'Neill, nurse practitioner and vice chair of the University of Southern California's Department of Nursing

CHAPTER ONE

Serving Humanity

Jim Delgado was a patient in the COVID-19 unit of a Washington, DC, hospital. Because of the virus's highly contagious nature, he, like all COVID-19 patients, was not allowed any visitors. Besides being very ill, Jim felt alone, hopeless, and scared. His nurses, like millions of nurses caring for COVID-19 victims all over the world, went out of their way to make him feel less isolated. Besides monitoring his vital signs and administering treatments, they sat at his bedside, held his hand, and offered him words of encouragement. Even after working twelve-hour shifts, they stopped in, on their own time, to check on him before heading home. They became his support system, filling in for his loved ones who could not be with him. Delgado recalls:

> At my worst, at my darkest hours, these three nurses provided actual family care. The human touch they provided was most comforting. I felt as if my family was there holding my hand, stroking my head, their gentle touch on my back, words of encouragement, and much much more. . . . I'm without words on how grateful I am to these nurses who made me feel so hopeful so less alone.[3]

Like Delgado, millions of COVID-19 survivors are extremely grateful to nurses, physicians, and other health care professionals for giving them the emotional support they needed to fight and defeat the virus. Even in fatal cases, lots of families have credited health care professionals for helping ease their loved one's passing. Many nurses have made it their mission to stay with end-of-life patients as they passed on. Others have used their personal cell phones so that dying patients could FaceTime with their families. This small caring act has allowed patients and their loved ones to see each other one last time, exchange words of love, and say their final good-byes.

Throughout the pandemic, health care professionals have gone beyond their job description in the service of others—often under horrible circumstances. They have frequently worked around-the-clock in overcrowded and inadequately staffed hospitals. Many have done so without sufficient medical supplies or personal protective equipment (PPE). Some have witnessed more pain, suffering, and death than they ever imagined. At the height of the pandemic in New York City, for example, more than seven hundred COVID-19 deaths occurred in just one day.

Not surprisingly, large numbers of health care workers have contracted the virus, some fatally. But no matter the circumstances and the risks, these stalwart individuals have consistently and selflessly put the needs of others above their own. As Dennis Canale, a New York physician assistant, explains, "The most impressive thing that I see is the staff I work with. . . . They didn't take that job thinking, 'Hey, I'm going to go out today and put my life on the line.' . . . But they're all there doing it. It's amazing to watch."[4]

> "The most impressive thing that I see is the staff I work with. . . . They didn't take that job thinking, 'Hey, I'm going to go out today and put my life on the line.' . . . But they're all there doing it."[4]
>
> —Dennis Canale, physician assistant

Facing Poor Working Conditions

In normal times, most hospitals have enough staff, beds, and intensive care units (ICUs) to care for sick patients. However, during the height of the pandemic in the spring of 2020, the huge volume of COVID-19 patients overwhelmed health care facilities.

Many lacked enough rooms, beds, ICUs, and medical equipment to handle the flood of patients. In some hospitals, beds lined hallways, and operating rooms, storage rooms, and other underused areas of hospitals were transformed into COVID-19 wards. When these became full, tents, modified shipping containers, ships, and convention centers were converted into field hospitals. Nor was it unusual for health care professionals to be involved in setting up these makeshift units. Atlanta nurse Jeanine Wright, for instance, gave up her day off to help members of her hospital's staff transform several operating rooms into ICUs for COVID-19 patients.

Not only was space at a minimum, the large number of severely ill patients who needed specialized care stretched hospital staffs. Nurses, doctors, respiratory therapists, and other health care professionals willingly worked extremely long hours without a break, seven days a week. This is how KP Mendoza, a New York City ICU nurse, described his experience in April 2020: "I want people to know that this is beyond difficult. . . . I run around for twelve hours a day, sometimes more if it was particularly busy that

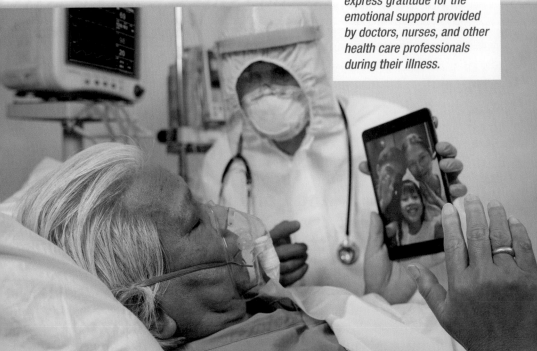

A medical worker helps a patient use a tablet to visit with her loved ones in a video call. Patients who have recovered from COVID-19 express gratitude for the emotional support provided by doctors, nurses, and other health care professionals during their illness.

shift. Nowadays, I consider myself lucky if I have time to eat, blessed if I have time to pee more than once a shift."[5]

The demand for health care professionals was so great that thousands of older nurses and physicians delayed their retirement or voluntarily came out of retirement to treat COVID-19 patients. Their actions were especially altruistic, since studies suggest that older people are at a greater risk of contracting a severe case of COVID-19 than younger individuals. Sixty-six-year-old Stanley Berry, a Michigan physician, was one of these vulnerable volunteers. "I didn't take this decision lightly," he explained. "This could be the last thing I do on earth, but I felt very strongly about it. . . . I don't want to die, and I'm not in this to be a hero, but medicine's been good to me and the city of Detroit's been good to me, and we're being clobbered right now. My will is made, so I'm just going to try to . . . help."[6]

Other health care professionals made sacrifices, too. Many of those who normally worked in other departments willingly redeployed to emergency rooms, ICUs, and COVID-19 units, where the need and the danger were greatest. Some traveled across the country, as well as to other countries, to lend a hand. Spikes in cases occurred in different regions at different times. Thousands of nurses who resided in areas that were not hard hit (at the time) flocked to understaffed pandemic hot spots, even though the move took them away from their homes and families for extended periods and exposed them to the virus. Nichole Imhoff was one of these nurses. The Michigan nurse spent six weeks separated from her husband and two children while caring for COVID-19 patients in the Bronx in the spring of 2020. "I was scared every single day," she says. "When I first got there, I was literally scared to breathe the air around me."[7] Nevertheless, like so many others, she ignored her fear so that she could help.

> "I run around for twelve hours a day, sometimes more if it was particularly busy that shift. Nowadays, I consider myself lucky if I have time to eat, blessed if I have time to pee more than once a shift."[5]
>
> —KP Mendoza, registered nurse

The Challenge of Inadequate Equipment and Supplies

Lack of PPE has also raised health care providers' fears. Even under ordinary circumstances, health care professionals risk exposure to infectious diseases. The risk has skyrocketed during the pandemic. The new coronavirus is a highly contagious airborne pathogen. It mainly spreads when people inhale respiratory droplets that infected people shed when they cough, sneeze, or talk. Moreover, infected droplets can settle on a person's clothes, on shoes, and on hard surfaces and remain infectious anywhere from one hour to five days, depending on the surface. Touching these viral droplets then touching one's mouth or nose can also make a person sick.

To protect themselves and those they come in contact with, health care professionals don PPE whenever they treat patients with infectious illnesses. This equipment includes face shields, gloves, goggles, head coverings, long-sleeved gowns, and N95 masks, which are special masks that filter out 95 percent of airborne particles. Most protective gear is designed to be discarded once it is used or exposed to a contagious patient. However, due to the vast numbers of COVID-19 patients, the demand for these items has far exceeded the supply. In fact, according to the World Health Organization, during some periods the worldwide demand for masks has been one hundred times greater than normal. In fact, in April 2020 the US government reported that the national stockpile of PPE was down by 90 percent. As a result, many health care professionals were forced to reuse their PPE. This significantly reduced or eliminated the equipment's effectiveness.

Early on, nurses and physicians often had to wear the same protective gear throughout a twelve-hour shift. Indeed, in a number of health care facilities, PPE was so scarce that some workers were given a single, one-time use, paper surgical mask to use for a week, or one disposable face shield to use indefinitely. In some cases health care providers resorted to makeshift equipment such

Brave Environmental Service Workers

Hospital environmental service workers are people who clean patients' rooms. Also known as housekeepers, these men and women are often low-paid people of color who lack employee benefits such as health insurance or paid sick leave. Moreover, because of shortages of protective gear, they have frequently worked without adequate PPE. According to Anita, a Baltimore environmental service worker:

> Before doctors and nurses can begin their work treating people receiving treatment for COVID-19, cleaners like me do the very hard and dangerous work of disinfecting and keeping every surface up to a critically safe standard. Our work is essential to reducing the spread of this disease and we are risking our lives every time we go to work, yet we receive no additional pay, benefits or protection.

> Yet these dedicated workers have not quit. In fact, many have not only cleaned rooms, they have spent extra time with COVID-19 patients, talking, joking, and praying with them. They have offered words of encouragement and listened when patients expressed their worries and fears. In fact, many patients have credited these workers with helping them get through the illness.

Quoted in CNN, "He Was a Covid-19 Patient. She Cleaned His Hospital Room. Their Unexpected Bond Saved His Life," KVIA, June 11, 2020. https://kvia.com.

as bandanas and homemade face coverings for masks and used black plastic trash bags for head coverings and gowns. Therefore, large numbers of health care professionals were practically unprotected. They faced prolonged exposure to the virus, and many became infected. The situation, according to Dr. Joseph Habboushe, a New York City emergency room physician, was "like sending a soldier into war where everyone else has armor and we don't have armor."[8] It would have been understandable if health care providers refused to work without adequate protection, but even in the worst of circumstances, they put their patients first.

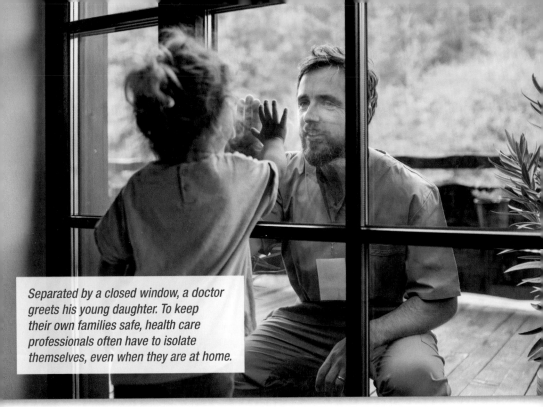

Protecting Loved Ones

Throughout the pandemic health care professionals have not only faced challenges at work, they have also had to worry about exposing their loved ones to the virus at the end of the work day. In order to avoid this, they have taken a number of measures. For instance, to keep their loved ones safe from being contaminated by viral droplets that may have settled on their clothes or bodies, many health care workers remove all their garments, put their clothes in the laundry, spray their shoes with disinfectant, and carefully shower before having any contact with their loved ones.

Some have taken more extreme measures. Such measures frequently involve health care workers giving up important aspects of their lives to protect their families. To keep their loved ones safe, some health care professionals isolate themselves within their homes. These individuals move into a separate part of the house from the rest of their family, even though doing so is difficult for them and their loved ones. Very young children, especially, have trouble understanding why their parent refuses to interact with them. Lauri Halbrook, a New Orleans nurse and mother of two young children, isolated herself in this way. She explains:

> It was heartbreaking because you can hear your children cry. You can hear them [testing] the lock on the door. And you can hear little footsteps, and it just breaks your heart because you want to be with them. I was trying to explain to a 3-year-old coronaviruses. And I was like, "You know there's a big germ that's out there that's hurting a lot of people, and I want to snuggle with you more than anything in the world right now, but Mommy can't sleep with you. I need to stay away to keep you safe."[9]

Other concerned health care workers have moved into garages and backyard tents. Some have avoided going home at all, temporarily living in hospital on-call rooms, hotels, or even in their

Applauding Health Care Professionals

When the COVID-19 pandemic began to surge throughout the world, most countries locked down, and people sheltered in place inside their homes. Health care workers did not have this option. They have put their own lives on the line every day. Their efforts did not go unnoticed or unappreciated. For weeks at a time, during the evening shift change when many health care workers entered and left hospitals, appreciative people leaned out of windows or stood on porches, balconies, fire escapes, and doorsteps and applauded.

This nightly ritual began in January 2020 in Wuhan, China, where the pandemic began. It later took off in Italy. As reports and videos of these events spread on social media, so did the reach. Before long people all over the world were participating. They cheered, clapped, whistled, banged pots, sang, and honked car horns every night in order to show their gratitude, appreciation, and respect for these dedicated caregivers.

These nightly ceremonies helped cheer up exhausted health care workers and lower their stress. It also allowed participants who were stuck at home to let off steam and interact with others in a safe manner.

cars. For example, Laura, an Oregon nurse, lived for a while in a pop-up truck camper in the parking lot of the hospital where she worked.

Emotional Trauma

The pressure and fear of keeping themselves and their loved ones safe have taken a toll on many health care workers, as have the horrors they have witnessed day after day. Even in the best of times, health care professionals experience emotional stress. To keep themselves emotionally healthy, they cannot let the pain and suffering they see affect them personally. However, the extreme conditions and trauma they have confronted during the pandemic have made this hard to do. As Mendoza explains:

> Even when I leave the hospital, I can't escape this plague. The Coronavirus follows me home literally and metaphorically. It's on the soles of my shoes, on my clothes as I strip bare at the door, and on my hands as I scrub them red and raw to rid myself of the feelings of filth and decay. It's in the sirens I hear outside wondering if that's the next victim of this virus, in the ping of a text from a coworker who is informing me that our colleague's father just died from COVID-19, and it's in the ventilator alarms that go off in my mind even when my apartment is desolately silent.[10]

Not surprisingly, many health care professionals have reported dealing with dark thoughts, nightmares, anxiety, depression, and symptoms of post-traumatic stress disorder. Some have had problems sleeping or eating properly. A July 2020 survey conducted by the American Nurses Foundation looked at how the pandemic affected the emotional health of nearly ten thousand nurses. Seventy-two percent of the respondents reported having sleep issues, and almost one-third reported dealing with symptoms of depression. Nevertheless, most health care professionals do not hesitate to care for the sick. And they do so without letting their own pain, fear,

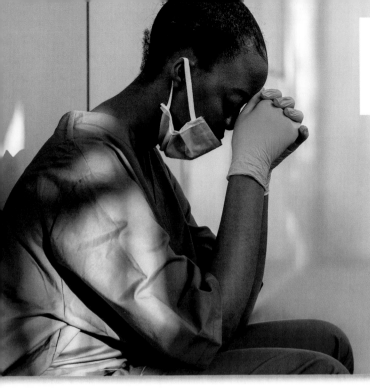

and anxiety show. As Wright explains, "When I go into that patient's room, they are looking to me for help. They look for comfort in me. If I freak out or show I have fear, I don't think that is very good. . . . When I go home, it's a different story. I am human."[11]

Paying the Ultimate Price

In March 2020 President Donald Trump referred to the battle against the COVID-19 pandemic as a war. During wars, there are always some brave troops who knowingly give up their own lives to save the lives of their comrades. Like these military heroes, many health care professionals have sacrificed their lives in the service of others. Knowing the danger they are in, some health care professionals have written or amended their wills and end-of-life wishes. Some of those with minor children have also made plans for their children's care in case of their own death. These actions are not over the top. As of May 2020, more than sixty-two thousand

"When I go into that patient's room, they are looking to me for help. They look for comfort in me. If I freak out or show I have fear, I don't think that is very good."[11]

—Jeannine Wright, registered nurse

health care workers in the United States had been infected with COVID-19. By August 2020, over nine hundred had lost their lives to the illness, according to a study sponsored by Kaiser Health News and the *Guardian*.

These warriors are of all ages and ethnicities. Some had existing health conditions that made them more vulnerable to contracting a severe case of COVID-19, including Matt Moeddel, a forty-three-year-old Cincinnati nurse. Moeddel, who lost his life to the virus in May 2020, was diabetic. Even though he was aware that this raised his risk level, he made it his mission to sit with and hold the hand of dying patients, until the coronavirus felled him.

Others, whose older age made them more vulnerable, also kept on working. Seventy-year-old Tomas Pattugalan, a Queens, New York, primary care physician, was among this group. According to his children, Pattugalan took the virus very seriously and was extremely careful to protect himself. But despite his best efforts, after two of his patients tested positive for COVID-19, he came down with it too. He died in March 2020, just five days after his diagnosis.

Young and healthy professionals were also struck down. California nurse Joshua Obra was only twenty-nine-years old when he succumbed to COVID-19 in July 2020. Tennessee nurse Neftali Rios was thirty-seven when his life was cut short by the coronavirus in April 2020. Rios collapsed in his home after being unable to catch his breath and died before emergency help arrived. Twenty-year-old California nursing assistant Valeria Viveros was another young victim. She lost her life to COVID-19 in April 2020. Besides working as a nursing assistant in a skilled nursing facility, she was studying to be a registered nurse. Unfortunately, she never got to achieve her goal.

Like these fallen warriors, during the COVID-19 pandemic, health care professionals have put themselves at risk on a daily basis. Few have backed down from the challenges and horrors they have faced, even if it led to their own deaths. These dedicated men and women have put aside their own fears and put the needs of others over their own, making them true heroes.

CHAPTER TWO

Keeping Society Safe and Functioning

During the pandemic many localities have mandated that people wear masks in public places. The practice, according to most health experts, helps protect the wearer from being infected by others and helps keep others from being infected by the wearer. Some people, however, feel that mask-wearing rules violate their personal freedom and have refused to wear one. This has sometimes led to violent confrontations between those opposed to wearing masks and workers responsible for enforcing the rules. For example, in July 2020 two men entered a New York City supermarket without any face coverings. When store employees asked the men to don masks, the men became irate. They went on a rampage, causing significant damage to the store and injuring eight store employees.

When these store employees hired on as grocery workers, they did not anticipate that working in a supermarket would endanger their lives. But that was before the COVID-19 pandemic struck. As essential workers, they have faced significant risk of being exposed to and contracting COVID-19. They have also faced threats from some angry members of the public. Yet despite the risk, they, like millions of other essential workers, have continued to report to work.

Essential workers are individuals who do jobs that involve keeping people and communities safe and society functioning. These individuals include but are not limited to first responders such as police, firefighters, and emergency medical technicians (EMTs); transportation and delivery workers; farmworkers and food processors; retail workers; and education professionals. The nature of their jobs puts them in close contact with many people each day, which has made them more vulnerable to contracting COVID-19. Large numbers of essential workers are people of color, who have disproportionately fallen ill and died from COVID-19. Their willingness to put their lives on the line during the pandemic has helped the rest of society run as normally as possible.

First Responders

First responders are among these heroes. When an emergency occurs, they are the first people on the scene. Even in normal times, they handle life-or-death situations and face danger. During the pandemic they have faced even greater risk. EMTs and firefighters have routinely answered 911 calls that put them in close physical contact with large numbers of people who either presented symptoms of COVID-19 or were asymptomatic but still infectious. Police officers have faced similar risk. They have entered homes to investigate at-home deaths, which may or may not have been caused by the coronavirus. They have come in face-to-face contact with people suspected of crimes. Plus, they have often dealt with unruly crowds in bars and house parties packed with maskless people, despite social distancing and masking orders. With the pandemic raging, the likelihood that some of these individuals were infected with the coronavirus was strong.

Moreover, the nature of their work has made it difficult for first responders to maintain social distancing. The enclosed space of an ambulance, for instance, prevents EMTs from physically distancing themselves from members of their team, as well as from patients they transport—even if the patient has COVID-19. Police officers face a similar problem inside closed police cars. In fact, by mid-April 2020 more than twenty-three hundred New York City police officers had contracted COVID-19, and twenty-nine had died from it. "I know I am going to get it," a New York police detective said at the time. "It's completely, utterly unavoidable. . . . But we have no choice, this is what we do."[12]

Indeed, even in the face of a killer virus, EMTs, firefighters, and police officers have shown more concern for protecting society and keeping it functioning than for their own well-being. New York City emergency medical service firefighter Sherry Singleton is one of these dedicated first responders. She explains, "A lot of people are running away from this and we're running towards it."[13]

Moving People and Supplies

Other essential workers also perform jobs that keep society from falling apart. These individuals move people and supplies. They make it possible for health care and other essential workers to

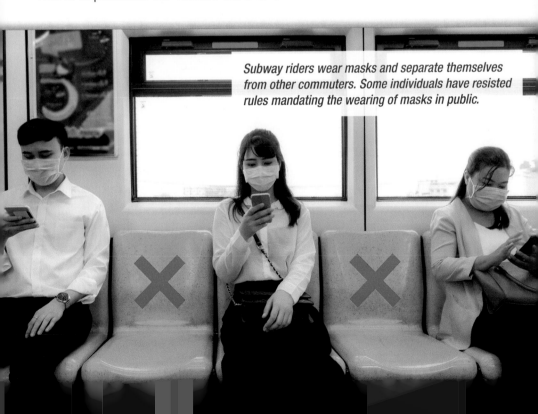

Subway riders wear masks and separate themselves from other commuters. Some individuals have resisted rules mandating the wearing of masks in public.

get to and from work. They also deliver mail and packages. And they transport food and essential items to hospitals, stores, and pharmacies. Although their work has raised their risk of exposure to the virus, many have put in very long hours to keep society and the economy running smoothly.

Bus drivers, as an example, have transported hundreds of passengers, including but not limited to health care professionals, first responders, and other individuals who may have been infectious. Passengers were not tested or questioned before boarding buses. In fact, people who suspected they were infected with COVID-19 sometimes traveled by mass transit to health care facilities to get tested or examined. Moreover, some cities have not imposed mask-wearing regulations or ridership limits on mass

Battling Wildfires During a Pandemic

As first responders, firefighters are at high risk of being exposed to COVID-19. Those who battle wildfires are especially vulnerable. Massive wildfires in California, Oregon, and other parts of the western United States between August and October required deployment of hundreds of firefighters. These men and women traveled from fire to fire, often in crowded fire helicopters, and often into areas where COVID-19 cases were surging, which raised their risk of contracting the coronavirus.

Fire crews also lived in close proximity to each other in base camps. They often stood elbow-to-elbow while fighting fires. Because they were in such close proximity to each other for long periods, if one member of a fire crew became infected, other members of the crew usually became infected, too. In fact, a study conducted by Colorado State University in the midst of the August 2020 wildfire season suggested that as many as 5 percent of wildfire crews would contract COVID-19 on the job, and 1 percent would lose their lives to it. As Mariana Ruiz-Temple, Oregon's chief deputy state fire marshal, explains, "The reality is you're going to see positives in camp, that's just the era we are in globally. Knowing that and not being afraid of that, is what's important."

Quoted in Miranda Green, "Federal Firefighter Units Juggle COVID-19 Infection on Fire Lines," NBC News, August 29, 2020. www.nbcnews.com.

transit, which has further increased a driver's chance of being exposed to the virus. In places that have had safety rules, it was usually up to bus drivers to enforce them, which sometimes led to conflicts. In an April 2020 incident in Columbus, Ohio, for example, an angry passenger who claimed to be infected with the coronavirus spat directly onto the bus driver's face. In other cases irate passengers purposefully coughed on drivers before disembarking.

Not surprisingly, many bus drivers have contracted COVID-19; by April, more than one hundred had lost their lives to it. Since that time, more have been infected and some have died. According to Seattle bus driver Kenneth Bryant, "The general public don't see it, but we're seeing members [of the Amalgamated Transit Union] dying all the time. We're putting our lives on the line getting in these buses."[14] Yet most bus drivers and other transit workers have continued to do their jobs. As a matter of fact, without the transportation they provide, many health care workers would not be able to do theirs.

Truck drivers, too, put themselves at risk to keep society functioning. By transporting essential supplies to stores and hospitals, they have ensured that the public has access to food, medicine, and other necessities. Many truckers have worked longer than normal hours under difficult circumstances. It has not been unusual for drivers who just finished a long haul to immediately set out again. Many have not gotten enough sleep or proper nutrition during their journeys. With truck stop and other roadside restaurants shuttered in the early months, getting a hot meal was difficult. And although drivers are alone in their vehicles much of the time, they come in contact with other drivers, truck stop attendants, and warehouse and store workers. These contacts have raised their risk of being exposed to the virus. Plus, they have often traveled to areas where the pandemic is surging. Crissy Becker, a truck driver from Maine, is one of these intrepid truckers. "I'm a mom," she writes. "Instead of going home, I stayed out driving my truck sometimes 24 hours at a time. . . . And there are

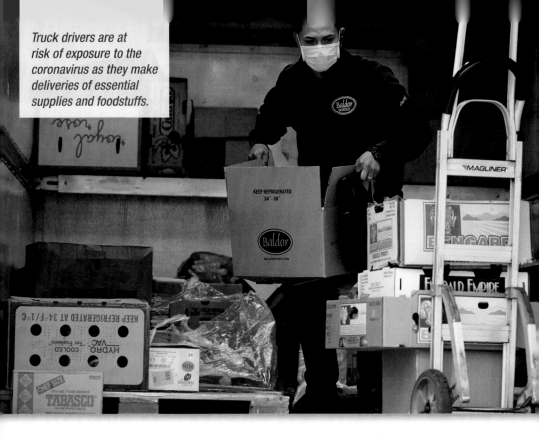

hundreds of thousands more like me . . . staying out here putting ourselves at risk of the COVID-19. So y'all can have what you need. . . . We are one of the only things keeping [the] economy as alive as it is."[15]

At-Risk Farmworkers and Food Processors

Before truck drivers can deliver food to businesses, farmworkers and food processors have to care for crops and livestock and must process and package meat, poultry, and produce. During the pandemic, many farmworkers and food processors have lacked personal protective gear. Moreover, they often work under cramped and crowded conditions, and many also live under these conditions. Their work and living environments have made them vulnerable to the virus. Nonetheless, these hard-working men and women have risked their health day after day so that food supply chains can remain open and the economy can keep moving.

Many farmworkers and food processors are immigrants who barely earn a living wage and who live in unhealthy, crowded spaces in which germs thrive. It is not unusual for groups of workers to live together and share beds in small, poorly ventilated

trailers and apartments. These conditions have made it almost impossible for individuals who tested positive for COVID-19 or who fell ill to self-quarantine. In May 2020 Armando Elenes, the secretary-treasurer of the United Farm Workers labor union, called these types of living quarters "ticking time bombs."[16]

Conditions in the fields are not much safer. Farmworkers frequently stand side by side planting and picking crops. When they take a break, they often congregate in whatever shade they can find. Few employers provide hand-washing stations or additional shaded spaces, which might have helped combat the spread of the virus.

Food processors have faced even more dangerous working conditions. The extremely close quarters in which they work have made them extremely vulnerable to becoming infected. They typically stand no more than 1 foot (30.5 cm) apart cutting and packaging meat, poultry, and produce during shifts that last ten to twelve hours. And they often lack face shields, masks, and gloves.

In the early months of the pandemic, meatpacking plants became COVID-19 hotbeds. Thousands of workers became infected, and some plants closed. Fearing long-term closures would wreck supply chains and cause food shortages, on April 28, 2020, Trump signed an executive order requiring meatpacking plants to continue operating despite the risk to workers. The order recommended but did not require that employers follow Centers for Disease Control and Prevention safety guidelines such as supplying workers with face coverings, increasing spacing in work areas, and performing COVID-19 testing and contact tracing of workers. However, many employers failed to follow these guidelines, and workers continued to become infected in record numbers. Rogelio Munoz Calderon was one of these workers. He worked in a meat-processing plant in Nebraska. Even though the coronavirus spread through his workplace and many of his peers got sick, Munoz Calderon kept going to work so that the public was supplied with meat. In August 2020 he lost his life to the virus. Many other workers in industries that supply food shared his fate. According to a report by Senator Elizabeth Warren, by mid-July 2020, thirty-six thousand meat-processing workers had contracted COVID-19, and more than one hundred had died.

Brave Retail Workers

Other brave essential workers have also put themselves in the line of fire to ensure others have food and basic necessities. Grocery workers, many of whom are teenagers, are among them. While most, but not all, states ordered nonessential businesses to shut down in the early months of the pandemic, grocery stores remained open. The large number of customers and coworkers with whom grocery store employees come in contact on a daily basis has put them at high risk of being exposed to the virus.

At the start of the pandemic, panic buying was widespread. Safety measures like social distancing and limits on the number of customers allowed in the store at one time were not yet enacted. Shoppers mobbed grocery stores, piling shopping carts with food and essential items so that they could shelter in place or self-quarantine if necessary. Grocery workers came in face-to-face contact with hundreds of people daily. And cashiers scanned and bagged thousands of items that had been touched, and possibly coughed on, by customers and other employees who may have been infectious. To accommodate all these shoppers, many clerks and cashiers worked twelve to fifteen hours a day. Plus, until mask wearing was mandated by state or local governments, some employers did not provide workers with PPE. In fact, some discouraged workers from wearing masks. As a result of all these challenges, workers were frequently exposed to the virus. "Whenever we open up the doors, it seems like it's Black Friday at a

The Violent Reaction to Mask Mandates

In May 2020 a security guard at a Michigan store was fatally shot when he asked a customer to don a mask. He is not the only essential worker who has been attacked (or threatened) over attempts to enforce a policy that has been shown to help protect people from coronavirus infection. Similar attacks and threats by people who oppose mask mandates have been reported at fast-food and other restaurants, big box retailers, and grocery stores around the country.

These individuals contend that mask mandates violate their civil liberties. Many have followed the lead of President Donald Trump, who has frequently disparaged the value of masks and only rarely has been seen wearing one in public. While the president (who contracted the virus in October) has not urged his followers to commit violence, he has made mask wearing a political issue. In a June 2020 *Wall Street Journal* interview, Trump said he believes that people who wear masks are showing their disapproval of him rather than trying to prevent the virus's spread. And, during the 2020 presidential campaign, he repeatedly mocked his opponent, Joe Biden, for wearing one.

clothing store," Aidan Gertson, an eighteen-year-old Georgia grocery clerk, explained at the time. "People swarm in. They try to get whatever they can before it's off the shelves. Every day. . . . It can be a little bit scary sometimes because you never know if these customers have been exposed to the coronavirus. You don't know if they're bringing it in with them."[17]

As the pandemic progressed, most supermarket chains began to implement safety measures to help protect customers and workers. To make sure these measures are followed, grocery store workers have been given the additional duties of sanitizing checkout counters and shopping carts and enforcing mask wearing, item limits, and social distancing rules. They also have been responsible for getting rid of used gloves, masks, and sanitizing wipes that inconsiderate customers have left in shopping carts, which has further raised workers' chances of becoming infected.

Not surprisingly, by mid-April 2020 the United Food and Commercial Workers International Union reported that at least three thousand grocery workers had contracted COVID-19, and more than forty had died from it. Nevertheless, grocery workers have risked their own safety and well-being to keep people supplied with food and basic necessities, the economy moving, and society functioning. And they have done so even though wages for most grocery workers are low. New York grocery clerk Wally Waugh is one of these unsung heroes. "I'm very proud to be a grocery store worker," he says. "Some of us were working 15-hour days. We knew we had to stay, and we did. People still have to eat. . . . I don't see myself as a hero. I see myself doing a job that's needed. As long as I can do it, and I'm not sick, I'm going to do it."[18]

Tending to the Needs of Children

Educating and supporting children is essential to society. Most schools were shuttered in the spring and in-person classes were canceled. Since that time, some schools have reopened for in-person teaching, some have continued with distance learning, and others have used a mix of both. Throughout this time, teachers, school bus drivers, food service workers, and other school employees have not been idle. They have made sure that students continued to be educated, supported, and fed.

With little advanced notice, teachers went from being in-person instructors to online instructors. Although online learning has received a lot of criticism for a number of good reasons, this does not detract from the efforts made by many dedicated teachers. They spent a lot of time developing lessons and materials in new virtual formats. They also created individualized paper learning packets for students who lacked internet access. Some teachers took it upon themselves to drop off and pick up these packets at each student's

CHAPTER THREE

Turning the Tide

Soon after COVID-19 became a threat to world health, a group of scientists at the University of California, San Francisco, teamed up to study how the new coronavirus interacts with human cells, and then to test whether any existing antiviral drugs, singularly or in combination, might disable the virus's effect on the cells. The scientists have worked around the clock in hopes that they might discover a way to effectively treat COVID-19. As news of their work became known, an international team of scientists representing laboratories throughout the world joined the research team. Their work is ongoing. It has led to a number of new discoveries that may help control the ability of the virus to take over cells, replicate, and spread throughout the body.

These scientists are just a few of the many dedicated individuals who have waged war against the coronavirus. Public health professionals and scientists, as well as many unsung heroes, have worked diligently to end or at least slow the pandemic. Some have focused on guiding the public's response to the pandemic. Others have turned their attention to protecting the most vulnerable members of society. Still others have worked to develop effective treatments and vaccines.

Public Health Warriors

Public health officials have been in the forefront of the battle. On any given day these doctors, nurses, scientists, and lab technicians can be found monitoring disease outbreaks and compiling and analyzing data related to these outbreaks.

Using this data, they develop public health policies and communicate information to government officials and the general public. Their work helps guide the public's response to disease. These dedicated professionals have worked especially hard during the pandemic. For example, the former director of Ohio's Department of Health, Dr. Amy Acton, started her workday at 4:00 a.m. and worked until late into the night gathering information about the coronavirus, which she used to guide her state's response to the pandemic. Largely due to her recommendations, Ohio was one of the first states to issue social distancing guidelines, limit the number of people at social gatherings, and shut down nonessential businesses. And while the president held televised briefings to report on the fight against the virus, Acton held daily briefings too. She did not sugarcoat the facts. Instead, in a calm and reassuring manner, she presented accurate details about the virus's symptoms and virulence, as well as information about testing, quarantining, and what safety measures Ohioans needed to follow to keep each other safe. She explains, "I really believe that people, when given the information, will use that to help themselves feel prepared. I'm a person who likes to know the reality."[21]

Indeed, many Americans have been confused by mixed messages. On the one hand, they have seen televised images of horribly overcrowded hospitals and dying patients or read accounts of people who were suffering from the disease and, often, dying alone. On the other hand, the public has also heard optimistic statements and messages from the president and some other conservative politicians. Accurate information presented by local, state, and national public health officials has helped ease this confusion. Dr. Anthony Fauci, the director of the National Institute of Allergy and Infectious Diseases, has been the face of the government's response concerning COVID-19. Like hundreds of other public health experts, Fauci has worked about eighteen hours a day to help steer the public's response to the pandemic.

Despite their dedication, some public health officials have faced attacks on their competence and character by protesters and politicians opposed to safety policies that the officials helped

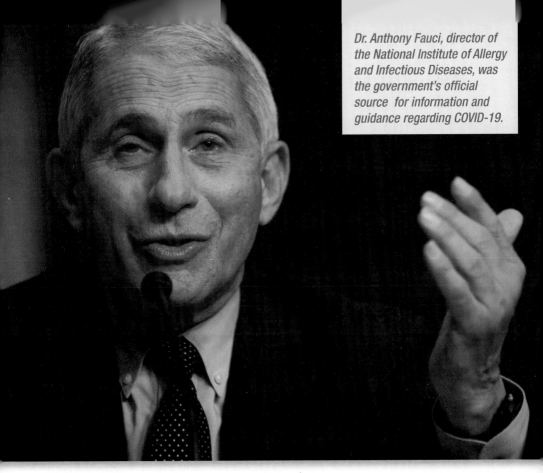

enact, such as mask wearing and stay-at-home orders. Some, like Acton, have faced verbal abuse and physical threats. She stepped down from her directorship position in June 2020 but took on a new role in which she has helped Ohioans prepare to deal with possible future conditions of the pandemic. Similarly, Fauci has received death threats, which led to him being assigned a bodyguard. Yet in spite of pushback against them, public health officials have devoted themselves to keeping the virus from spreading. As Lauri Jones, the county health director of Okanogan County, Washington, insists, "I am not going to back down from this, regardless of any threats. We'll continue to do our jobs. This isn't a short-term virus."[22]

> "I am not going to back down from this, regardless of any threats. We'll continue to do our jobs. This isn't a short-term virus."[22]
>
> —Lauri Jones, county health director of Okanogan County, Washington

Protecting the Homeless

Through analyzing data about COVID-19, public health professionals have identified several groups that have been disproportionately affected by the coronavirus. These include the elderly and chronically ill, the homeless, the poor, and frontline workers. Some selfless individuals have made it their mission to serve and protect these vulnerable groups, even though doing so raises their own risk of falling ill. Through their actions they have helped slow the spread of the virus.

Homeless populations are among the vulnerable groups they have targeted. People living in homeless shelters and out on the street face a high risk of being exposed to the coronavirus and of transmitting it to others. Homeless shelters are typically crowded places where social distancing is difficult. In this type of congregate environment, germs spread rapidly; one carrier could easily infect multiple people who then go on to infect others.

Stopping the Spread in the Americas

Maria Pia Sanchez is a Chilean interior designer who lives in Florida. Wanting to help lessen the spread of COVID-19 in Florida, in March 2020 she and a few of her friends began making face masks for local frontline workers.

Sanchez was also concerned about people back home in Chile and other parts of Latin America. She knew that many people would not have access to masks. So, she created a Facebook Group page called Por Todas Masks Initiative. Through the page, she enlisted six hundred volunteer mask makers, many of whom were from Central and South America.

To help and instruct the volunteers, Sanchez posted videos and patterns on the group page. She even came up with special designs for waterproof masks and masks for children with Down Syndrome. Although the group's goal was to make and donate seven thousand masks, by August 2020, Por Todos Masks Initiative, had made and donated fourteen thousand masks in the United States and Latin America.

Life on the street is even riskier. During the pandemic some homeless shelters have shut down completely, while others have set limits on the number of people they serve. This has caused a lot of homeless people to camp on the street, where they lack adequate access to food, drinking water, sanitation and hygiene facilities, protection from the weather, and connections to social services and health care. Nor do many have face masks. Plus, those who suspect they are infected have no real way to self-quarantine. "A shelter-in-place order works great if you have a home," explains Martha Stone, director of Cross Roads House, a New Hampshire homeless shelter. "But if you're home-less, it presents significant challenges."[23] All these conditions have made homeless individuals vulnerable to infection by the virus and spreading it among themselves, as well as among members of the general population with whom they come in contact.

"A shelter-in-place order works great if you have a home. But if you're homeless, it presents significant challenges."[23]

—Martha Stone, director of Cross Roads House, a New Hampshire homeless shelter

Social workers, public health professionals, and other individuals have helped lessen this threat. In California, Florida, New Hampshire, New York, and Texas, among other places, volunteers, social workers, and city and county employees have set up isolation sites in hotels where infected homeless individuals could self-quarantine. In Florida's Miami-Dade County, county employees have erected hand-washing stations on the streets and distributed hand sanitizer and COVID-19 information sheets to homeless people. Some have monitored homeless individuals' temperature (because fever is one symptom of COVID).

Across the country in Redondo Beach, California, Xan Wesley, a recent high school graduate and an EMT, administered COVID-19 tests to people in homeless encampments. Other individuals have also stepped up to help, like Hartford, Connecticut, police officer Jim Barrett. He has spent his free time distributing donated shoes, clothing, and food to the homeless. Shaun

Griffin is one of the people Barrett has helped. "I see him out here all times of day and night. . . . If it was up to me he'd get a Nobel Peace Prize,"[24] Griffin says.

Even though Barrett is not likely to win the Nobel Prize, his actions and the actions of other brave and unselfish individuals have helped protect vulnerable homeless people. These unsung heroes have put themselves at risk in order to lessen the risk to others.

Helping Tribal Communities

According to public health data, people living in disadvantaged communities have been disproportionately infected by coronavirus. Many individuals in this group are impoverished people of color. Members of the Navajo Nation, in particular, have been hard hit. The Navajo Nation encompasses about 16 million acres (6.5 million ha) across parts of New Mexico, Arizona, and Utah. It is the largest Indian reservation, in total land area, in the United States. About 173,600 people live on the reservation, often under conditions that can negatively impact a person's health. For instance, it is not unusual for multigenerational Navajo families to live in crowded homes, where germs can be passed around easily. This has increased members of these households' chances of coming down with COVID-19.

Adding to the problem, approximately 30 to 40 percent of Navajo homes lack indoor plumbing and access to clean running water. This makes hand washing and other forms of sanitation that can destroy the coronavirus problematic. Because the reservation is so spread out, some residents travel miles to community wells to get clean water. They often wait in long lines at the wells and then have to haul the water home. This has made social distancing and sheltering in place during the pandemic all the more challenging. To minimize trips out of their homes, people have used what little water they have sparingly, which is especially dangerous during a time when hand washing is vital. George McGraw, the founder of DigDeep, a nonprofit group that deals with water access, explains, "When it comes to COVID-19, all we have is prevention. We have no treatment, no vaccine. You can do two

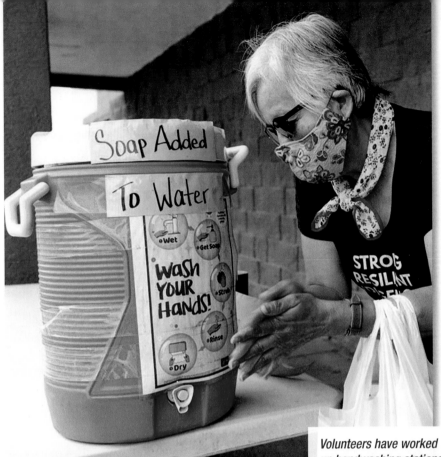

Volunteers have worked to set up handwashing stations in remote villages in the Navajo Nation. Efforts such as this have helped reduce COVID-19 cases and deaths among the underserved Navajo.

things—wash your hands frequently and you can isolate yourself from other people. Neither is possible if you don't have running water at home."[25]

Adding to the problem, more than half of the members of the Navajo Nation live below the poverty line. Many are food insecure and have underlying health conditions like diabetes and heart disease, which worsens their prognosis if they become infected. All of these factors have made members of the Navajo Nation susceptible to contracting and dying of COVID-19. According to an ABC News report, as of May 2020, the Navajo Nation had experienced the highest infection rate per capita in the United States.

Many individuals have dedicated themselves to controlling and preventing the spread of the infection among tribal members. Jonathan Nez, the president of the Navajo Nation, is among these

Stopping Evictions

Millions of people lost their jobs during the COVID-19 pandemic. Some lacked sufficient funds to pay rent and, therefore, faced eviction. Without sufficient funds and nowhere to go, many of these people confronted the real threat of becoming homeless, which would have increased their risk of contracting and spreading the virus. Mario Salerno, a landlord, who owns eighteen apartment buildings in Brooklyn, New York, did not want this to happen to his approximately three hundred tenants. Therefore, he waived all April 2020 rents.

Because of his caring act, Salerno lost thousands of dollars in rent payments. And, he still had to pay water, utility, and tax bills. Yet, he was more interested in lessening his tenants' stress and keeping the community safe, than in his own losses. "My concern is everyone's health," he explained. "I told them [the tenants] just to look out for your neighbor and make sure that everyone has food on their table."

Quoted in Matthew Haag, "This Brooklyn Landlord Just Canceled Rent for Hundreds of Tenants," *New York Times*, April 3, 2020. www.nytimes.com.

people. In addition to his administrative duties as the president of a sovereign nation, he has spent almost every day driving across the huge reservation hauling water, firewood, cleaning supplies, and food to residents. Other individuals, like Sam Bryant, who works for a local social service agency, have delivered boxes of donated food, water, and hand sanitizer to people living in the most isolated parts of the reservation. Community health workers have traveled throughout Navajo lands checking on sick individuals; while volunteers and staff members of various nonprofit agencies have built and set up hand-washing stations in Navajo villages. Others, like Linda Myers, the founder of Adopt-A-Native-Elder, a nonprofit organization that helps poor tribal elders, have worked with donors and volunteers to deliver food, face masks, water, and other supplies to elderly Navajo. Many other people also pitched in. Through their efforts, COVID-19 cases and deaths among Navajo decreased considerably. As Myers explains, "The biggest thing is that people have stepped up. . . . It's really made a difference."[26]

Devoted Caregivers

Many other selfless individuals have also stepped up to help vulnerable populations. Home aides who care for homebound elderly, disabled, and chronically ill people are among these often unacknowledged heroes. Home aides go to people's homes, where they help clients dress, bathe, groom, prepare meals, and shop, among other duties. They also provide clients with companionship. In addition, they go with their clients to doctor appointments, and some provide medical services. Without these caregivers, many sick, disabled, and elderly people would be forced to go to overcrowded hospitals and nursing homes for care—places where they are more likely to be exposed to the coronavirus. Moreover, since aging weakens the immune system, once exposed, elderly people are more likely than younger individuals to develop a severe case of COVID-19.

Many home aides are low-paid women of color. A large number do not have cars and routinely use public transportation to get to and from their clients' homes, a situation that increases their own chances of being exposed to the coronavirus. Rashida Ahmed cared for an elderly woman in the New York area. To get to the woman's home, Ahmed depended on public transportation. In March 2020 Ahmed fell ill with COVID-19. She lost her life to the illness within a month. Her family is unsure whether she became infected during her daily commute or in the course of her work. Yet knowing the risk, she, like many other dedicated home aides, refused to abandon her client.

Daily commutes have not been the only risk home aides have faced. It is almost impossible for home aides to physically distance themselves from their clients. Bathing, dressing, grooming, and feeding another person involves close physical contact. And due to shortages, many home aides have not been issued medically approved masks or other PPE. Some have used homemade cloth masks, and some have resorted to cutting up plastic soda bottles to use as face shields. Plus, they have also faced the risk of bringing the virus home to their families. Nevertheless, these brave and dedicated individuals have persevered. Stacey D. is one of these devoted home aides. "I made the choice years ago that this is what I wanted to do," she explains. "But I pray each morning before I come out, take the necessary precautions, and leave it at that. What are you going to do, run away? You can't do that."[27]

Toiling in Laboratories

While public health professionals, social workers, home aides, and other dedicated individuals have worked tirelessly to mitigate the spread of the virus and to protect the most vulnerable members of society, scientists and technicians have toiled in laboratories. They have been focused on developing vaccines that could provide some degree of immunity against the coronavirus. Others have worked to find treatments that would lessen the severity of the illness, leading to fewer deaths.

These researchers have been working at a feverish pace. Typically, developing a vaccine or a new drug takes three to five years. However, almost as soon as the new coronavirus emerged, scientists all over the world dropped their existing research and turned their full attention to COVID-19. Public and private institutes, academic groups, pharmaceutical companies, and research centers have formed national and international partnerships in an attempt to speedily end the pandemic. Operation Warp Speed, for example, is a collaboration between the US Department of Health and Human Services, other government agencies, and the private sector. Its aim is to fast-track the development and production of a vaccine. As an Operation Warp Speed partner, the National Institutes of Health (NIH) has teamed up with eighteen pharmaceutical companies. As Dr. Francis Collins, NIH director, explains, "In my 27 years at NIH,

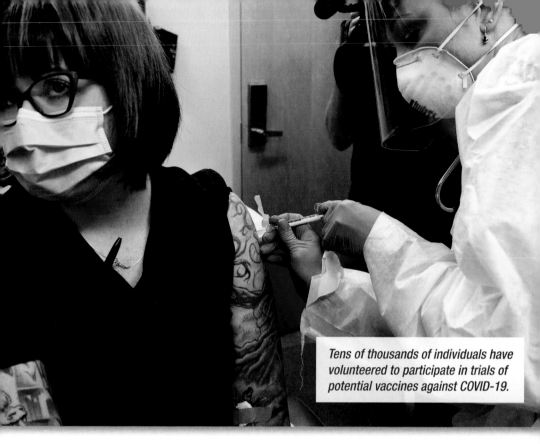

Tens of thousands of individuals have volunteered to participate in trials of potential vaccines against COVID-19.

I've never seen anything quite like this. There's been a willingness among people to set aside all kinds of other concerns. They've gathered around the same table, worked on vaccine design and implementation, and gotten out there in the real world to launch clinical trials."[28]

Worldwide about one hundred companies have been focused on creating a vaccine. Scientists have worked day and night, studying the virus, creating possible vaccines, and then testing the mixtures on cells and laboratory animals. In just a matter of months, dozens of potential vaccine candidates went into clinical trials.

In clinical trials, promising drugs and vaccines are tested for safety and efficacy on human subjects. Despite the possibility

"There's been a willingness among people to set aside all kinds of other concerns. They've gathered around the same table, worked on vaccine design and implementation, and gotten out there in the real world to launch clinical trials."[28]

—Dr. Francis Collins, director of the National Institutes of Health

that potential vaccines could cause a severe reaction, tens of thousands of brave individuals all over the world have volunteered to be test subjects. They have done so for many reasons. Some felt it was their civic duty to participate. Some stepped up in hopes that their efforts would help protect vulnerable people in the future. Others, like Jarelle Marshall of Cincinnati, wanted to set a good example for their children. "I always tell my son that what matters is what you do when people aren't looking,"[29] he explains.

No matter their reasons, it is clear that during a time when the world has needed ordinary people to step up and help stem the tide, scientists, public health experts, social service professionals, home aides, and thousands of volunteers have heeded the call. And their efforts have made a difference.

CHAPTER FOUR

Young Heroes

Bryce Rose is a Florida teen. In March 2020 when the high school she attended shut down due to COVID-19, she felt isolated and lonely. So did many of the residents of a local senior citizen community who were sheltering in place and therefore had little contact with each other or their loved ones. Rose wanted to do something to cheer up these lonely people. So she wrote and illustrated hundreds of letters and cards with messages of hope, which she taped to their apartment doors. "I told them that they are loved and that this will pass. I said that there's always a rainbow after the storm,"[30] she says.

Rose did not stop with these messages. There were lots more people in her community who needed cheering up, so she created thank-you cards for local frontline workers. By August 2020 she had made and distributed more than one thousand handmade cards and letters. The messages worked, brightening and cheering both Rose and those who received them. As she explains, "If you are feeling alone, then give back. It fills your heart."[31]

During the COVID-19 pandemic, many young people have performed large and small acts of kindness and generosity. They have helped get food to people in need; supported overworked and stressed frontline workers; gathered, created, and distributed PPE; and befriended lonesome children and senior citizens, among hundreds of other unselfish deeds. Their actions have made a positive impact on the lives of others.

Helping Health Care Professionals and First Responders

Health care workers, first responders, and essential workers have faced shortages of PPE from the start of the pandemic. A large number of young people have made it their mission to help solve this problem. Among these problem solvers is a group of Alpharetta, Georgia, high school seniors who love computer science. They created a computer program, which they call Project Paralink. It identifies health care institutions in need of specific equipment and suppliers that are willing to donate these items. The program also coordinates the delivery of the equipment through a network of young volunteer drivers.

One of the cofounders, Edward Aguilar, says the teens initially focused on collecting masks, gloves, sanitizing wipes, and cleaning supplies for local health care facilities. In just one day Paralink pinpointed which supplies area hospitals needed, located and contacted area businesses and residents who had stocked up on and were willing to donate these items, and arranged to have the supplies delivered to fifteen nearby hospitals.

In addition to these items, many of the health care facilities Paralink contacted needed face shields. So next the teens turned their attention to getting local and distant health care workers' these protective coverings. Using their computer program, they located traditional manufacturers willing to donate face shields. However, these donations were not adequate to fill the immense need. To augment the supply, the teens, with the help of fifty other maker spaces that Paralink found, began making face shields using 3-D printing technology. A network of about one thousand volunteer drivers picked up the shields and delivered them to health care facilities in seven states. On one occasion, Paralink set up a chain of volunteer drivers who transported face shields from Georgia to hospitals in New York State.

The teens did not neglect their home state, either. In June 2020, when new cases surged in Georgia, Paralink supplied an estimated 200,000 face shields within the state, half of which were 3-D

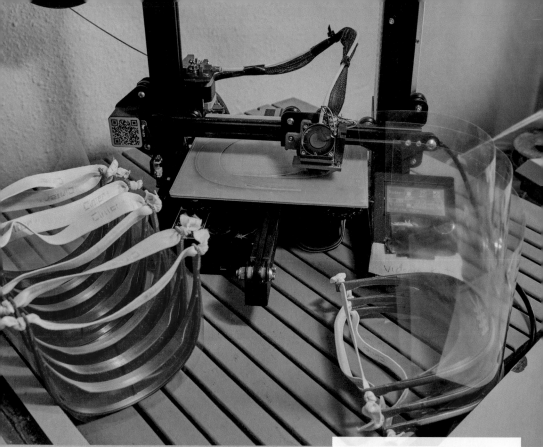

High school seniors in Georgia created a program called Project Paralink, which helped locate manufacturers willing to donate medical supplies. It identifies health care institutions in need of equipment and suppliers that are willing to donate these items. The teens, with the help of other makers that Paralink found, began making face shields using 3-D printing technology (shown here).

printed. In comparison, the Federal Emergency Management Agency supplied the state of Georgia with approximately 190,000 face shields, 10,000 fewer than the teens' contribution.

Project Paralink's creators are not alone in their efforts. Other young people have also taken on the challenge of providing frontline workers with PPE. In fact, hundreds of young people all over the United States have sewn, purchased, or collected thousands of face masks for health care and frontline workers. Angelina Lue, a California high school student, is one of these individuals. She started a GoFundMe campaign that raised $13,000 to buy face masks. By May 2020 Lue had purchased and donated more than fifteen thousand masks to San Francisco Bay Area and New York hospitals. Lue explains,

"I couldn't just sit back and watch what was going on. I felt like I had to do something to protect the people who are risking their lives and their families' lives. . . . It is important to know that everyone, especially we teenagers, can contribute."[32]

Making Masks a Priority

While many young people were busily getting PPE into the hands of frontline workers, others took it upon themselves to educate their peers about the importance of wearing a mask in public during the pandemic. A number of studies suggest that if 80 percent of the world's population wore masks during the pandemic, infection and death rates would be significantly lower. Artie Mendoza, a young Native American hip-hop musician who is also known as KiidTruth, has used music to get this message across to teenagers. He, along with other young tribal members of the Flathead Nation in Montana, released a video on social media in which they danced, sang, and rapped about the importance of mask wearing. In just the first four days that the video was posted, it received fifteen hundred views. The video, says fifteen-year-old Alishon Kelly, who lives on the Flathead Reservation, "is an excellent way to reach younger people. I've seen a lot of my peers posting it and watching it."[33]

Michelle Song, a San Francisco high school senior, had a similar idea. With the help of some friends, Song sewed and distributed free face masks to vulnerable populations throughout San Francisco. She also shipped more than five thousand homemade masks to homeless shelters and hospitals throughout the United States.

Although Song's efforts were extraordinary, she was not satisfied. Many people, including lots of young adults, do not understand how vital wearing a mask is in controlling the spread of the virus, and therefore they do not bother to wear a mask. So in

"I couldn't just sit back and watch what was going on. I felt like I had to do something to protect the people who are risking their lives and their families' lives."[32]

—Angelina Lue, California high school student

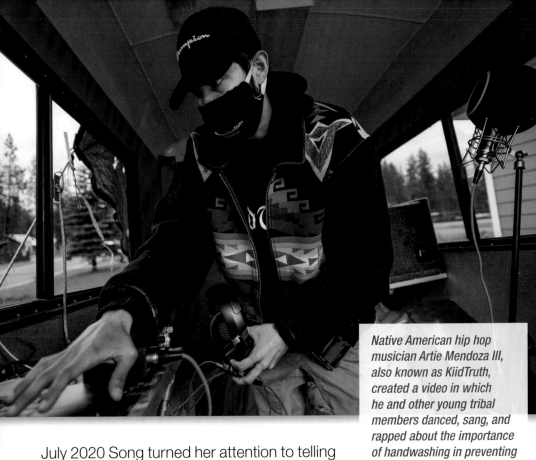

Native American hip hop musician Artie Mendoza III, also known as KiidTruth, created a video in which he and other young tribal members danced, sang, and rapped about the importance of handwashing in preventing the spread of COVID-19.

July 2020 Song turned her attention to telling other teens about the importance of mask wearing. She went online and gave talks and posted photos that promoted mask wearing. Song thinks that her campaign, as well as those of others like her, has made a positive impact. She believes that young people can be a driving force in changing society for the better.

Feeding People in Need

Other teens have made an extraordinary effort to supply hungry people with food. During the pandemic, many businesses have shut down, and large numbers of people have lost their primary source of income. Some individuals have had difficulty affording food, and food insecurity rates have shot up. According to a CBS News report, as of July 21, 2020, more than one in ten Americans did not have enough food. This was double the number of those lacking adequate food before the pandemic.

Drive By Heroes

Three Pearland, Texas, teenagers found a way to brighten the spirits of children during the COVID-19 pandemic. Twins Isaiah and Stephan Torres and their friend Jasmine Saenz spent much of their summer dressed in superhero costumes. Through their newly created organization Drive By Heroes, they scheduled drive-by visits to the homes of about three hundred Pearland children. Wearing face coverings and practicing social distancing, they entertained at outdoor birthday celebrations. In exchange for the visits, the teens accepted food and monetary donations, which they donated to a local nonprofit organization.

By August 2020, in addition to visiting hundreds of homes, they had collected about 4,500 pounds (2,041 kg) of nonperishable food. In fact, Drive By Heroes became so popular that the teens have created a video series on social media. Dressed in costume, the teenage superheroes pose riddles, lead fun exercises, show videos submitted by children, and interview special guests. Asked about their work, Isaiah explained, "We're just teenagers and a lot of people don't see us as people who would be doing stuff like this right now. A lot of us do care though. We want to be able to help out."

Quoted in Emily Gianbalvo, "Texas Teenagers Dressed as Superheroes Visit Kids While Collecting Food Donations," *Washington Post*, August 17, 2020. www.washingtonpost.com.

Not wanting others to go hungry, some young people have raised money to help fund depleted food banks. Others have organized food drives. Still others have used their own personal funds to purchase food, which they distribute to needy individuals. In the summer of 2020 Crystal Russell, a sixteen-year-old Milwaukee resident, used the money she earned doing two jobs to help feed hungry children. She bought hot dogs, buns, chips, fruit, juice, water, and bubble gum, which she prepared, sacked, and passed out to two hundred needy Milwaukee families. "Young children depend on school lunches and . . . there's really no school going on," she explained. "So, I just decided to pass out hot dog meals!"[34]

Dallas sisters Bella and Riley Sauter had a related idea. The girls wanted to help hungry homeless people in their community. Using their own money, they bought the fixings for thirty peanut butter and jelly sandwiches, which they prepared and distributed. However, thirty sandwiches were not sufficient to feed the burgeoning homeless population. Therefore, the following week, Bella and Riley made and distributed one hundred sandwiches, plus chips and a drink.

Proud of their efforts, the girls' mother posted information on social media about what they were doing. In response to the post, individuals and local businesses started dropping off bags of food on the Sauters' doorstep. Soon the girls were preparing hundreds of meal bags, which they delivered to homeless individuals and homeless shelters twice a week.

The teens still wanted to do more. With their parents' help, they formed a nonprofit corporation called Feed the People. This has allowed them to receive large financial donations from big corporations. As a result, the girls have been able to feed thousands of homeless individuals and families. Moreover, in September 2020 the sisters expanded their activities. With the goal of providing Halloween costumes and candy for children whose families lost their homes during the pandemic, they organized a candy and costume drive. As Bella explains, "We never saw it getting this big. It's been a huge blessing that it has. We've been able to help so many people. As long as we can, we'll do our part."[35]

Connecting People

Other young people have done their part by helping older people who were sheltering in place connect with their families, friends, and the outside world. Approximately 27 percent of Americans over age sixty live alone. As COVID-19 cases spread and cities issued stay-at-home orders in the spring, many older individuals felt cut off from their loved ones and society at large. Jordan Mittler, a sixteen-year-old New Yorker, has used technology to help some of these elderly people. Before the pandemic, he taught free weekly in-person technology classes to local senior citizens using a curriculum that he created. Once the lockdowns began, Mittler's students could no longer attend these classes. This did not deter Mittler. He believed his students needed technology more than ever to open up their world. Therefore, he decided to continue offering the weekly class via Zoom. It took him about a week of countless phone calls and texts to get all his students set up on the app and comfortable enough with it to sign on to his class. Before the first virtual class, Mittler amended his curriculum to help his students acquire technology skills relevant to life during the pandemic. For instance, he showed them how to grocery shop and bank online, how to use FaceTime and WhatsApp to visit with their grandchildren, how to access reliable COVID-19 news, and how to play online games, among other things that had become part of the new normal.

> "It's really up to our generation who know everything about technology and who [have] really been born into it to help the seniors who missed this entire technology boom."[36]
>
> —Jordan Mittler, New York high school student

The class has been so successful that Mittler, with the help of a few friends, has opened it up to any older person who wants to join. He has streamed every class on YouTube, hoping to help as many people as possible. He has added new classes, including one-on-one classes, question-and-answer sessions, and smartphone classes. In addition, he has started a teen ambassador program in which he enlists teen volunteers to locate and contact isolated seniors who might be interested in the classes. When asked about his efforts, the young instructor explained:

> Most of the seniors that I work with are retired and most live alone. I think almost all the seniors are staying in their homes right now, so the classes give them something to do every week. . . . It's really up to our generation who know everything about technology and who [have] really

been born into it to help the seniors who missed this entire technology boom and don't know how to communicate with friends and family in manners that we use every day and that we're so accustomed to.[36]

Other young people have taken a different tack. Five California teenagers, for instance, have also used technology to help ease isolated seniors' loneliness. They founded a free online service called COVID Networks. It has paired local high school student volunteers with residents of San Francisco Bay Area senior living facilities. The volunteers and the seniors are paired based on their having similar hobbies or interests. The young people have connected with their partners through frequent phone calls, Face-Time visits, and Zoom sessions. The teens have also organized

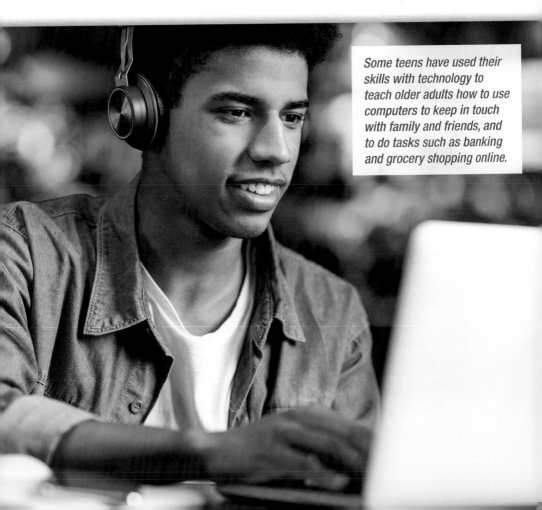

Some teens have used their skills with technology to teach older adults how to use computers to keep in touch with family and friends, and to do tasks such as banking and grocery shopping online.

fun games, led exercise classes, and gave music performances for their elderly friends on Zoom. Alex Wang, a cofounder of COVID Networks, explains:

> Many of us know grandparents in senior living communities who told us they were feeling lonely or isolated because they weren't able to receive physical visits and they didn't have any family who were contacting them virtually. . . . We thought that this was a great way we could help. Many high school students are sitting at home with a lot of time on their hands, so we thought this was a way to connect them with seniors to help give them someone to talk to.[37]

Everyday Acts of Kindness

While many young men and women have done tremendous things, thousands of others have performed small acts of kindness, which often go unrecognized but are heroic nonetheless. In every case, the young doers have put the needs of others above their own in this challenging time. A large number of young people, for example, have reached out to elderly and vulnerable neighbors at risk of contracting COVID-19. It is not unusual for teens to grocery shop for these individuals or to pick up and deliver groceries that a neighbor purchased online. Some teens have offered this help individually, while others have formed networks of shopping volunteers. Peyton LaFrenz, a Minneapolis high school junior, for example, started a free grocery shopping and delivery service for elderly neighbors. Individuals in need of groceries contact LaFrenz by email, then she or other teen volunteers telephone the individuals, get their shopping list, shop, and deliver the groceries to these people's doorsteps. LaFrenz explains, "I was kind of worried about them and how they were going to be able to be helped through this. It kind of turned into what can I do to help those that don't have relatives that live around here to do shopping for them."[38]

Special Masks for Special People

Many hearing-impaired people rely on lipreading to understand what people are saying. However, during the COVID-19 pandemic, when people began wearing masks that cover their mouths, it became very challenging for hearing-impaired people to communicate with others. As Karma Quick-Panwala, a severely hearing-impaired woman, explains, "I like to say lip reading is my superpower and masks are my kryptonite. I'm completely cut off from communication unless I have someone come speak to me personally so that I can lip read to understand what's being said."

Isabella Appell, a seventeen-year-old Californian, helped solve this problem. She started sewing and distributing traditional face masks at the beginning of the pandemic. When she learned about the challenges that hearing-impaired people faced, she created special masks with a clear plastic window over the wearer's mouth. To keep the clear plastic from fogging up when the wearer speaks, she sprayed the plastic with defogging spray. She called her project Talking Masks and set up website where people could obtain the masks free of charge. Appell gave any donations she received to charity.

Quoted in Leif Coorlim, "California Teen Is Sewing Masks That Help Hard-of-Hearing Read Lips," MSN, July 21, 2020. www.msn.com.

Other young people have let isolated neighbors know they care by surprising them with a pizza or other delivered meal. Some have left unsolicited care packages filled with essentials like toilet paper, tissues, and hand sanitizer at their neighbor's door or goodie bags loaded with homemade cookies, puzzle books, magazines, and other fun items. A group of elementary school children in Wildwood, New Jersey, found another way to lift their neighbors' spirits. In September 2020, they painted seashells with messages of hope and hid them all over the seaside community for others to find.

Other young people have spread kindness by offering help to families with children as well as reaching out to their own peers. Some teens have provided free babysitting services for the children of essential workers who were home alone due to school closures. Others have remotely tutored children having trouble with online lessons. They have helped with homework assignments and tried to make learning fun for children. Other young people have tried to brighten their own friends' spirits. One high school senior, as an example, organized a virtual prom for her classmates. Another set up a phone tree so that all her classmates could stay in touch with each other and no one would be left out.

> "It just feels really good to be able to help out the community in a time of crisis like this one, it all comes back to giving back."[39]
>
> —Peyton LaFrenz, Minneapolis high school student

These are just a few of the thousands of kind and compassionate acts that young people have performed. As LaFrenz explains, "It just feels really good to be able to help out the community in a time of crisis like this one, it all comes back to giving back."[39] Indeed, many ordinary people of all ages have helped out and given back to their communities during the COVID-19 pandemic. Whether their actions are large or small, they are all heroes.

Introduction: Ordinary People Doing Extraordinary Things

1. Quoted in Sari Harrar et al., "Our Challenge: A Million Gallons of Soup," *AARP Magazine*, June/July 2020, p. 65.
2. Quoted in Eric Lindberg, "These Skilled USC-Trained Nurse Practitioners Risk Their Health to Help Others," USC News, May 12, 2020. https://news.usc.edu.

Chapter One: Serving Humanity

3. Jim Delgado, "Thank You, Johns Hopkins Healthcare Heroes," Kudoboard, Johns Hopkins Medicine. www.kudoboard.com.
4. Quoted in Paul Moakley, "The Country Won't Work Without Them. 12 Stories of People Putting Their Lives on the Line to Help Others During Coronavirus," *Time*, April 9, 2020. https://time.com.
5. Quoted in Jason Kane, "Do Not Call Me a Hero," *PBS NewsHour*, April 24, 2020. www.pbs.org.
6. Quoted in Jamie Ducharme, "'This Could Be the Last Thing I Do on Earth.' A Michigan Doctor Was Going to Retire. Then Came the Coronavirus," *Time*, April 9, 2020. https://time.com.
7. Quoted in Leon Hendrix, "Rockford Nurse Who Fought COVID-19 in NYC: 'Very Humbling, Very Real,'" Wood TV, May 26, 2020. www.woodtv.com.
8. Quoted in Molly Kinder, "Meet the COVID-19 Frontline Heroes," Brookings Institution, 2020. www.brookings.edu.
9. Quoted in Katy Reckdahl, "As a Nurse, I Took an Oath to Take Care of People. But My Children and Husband Didn't Sign Up to Get Sick," *Time*, April 9, 2020. https://time.com.
10. Quoted in Kane, "Do Not Call Me a Hero."
11. Quoted in Joanne Vitelli, "Unsung Heroes of Georgia's COVID-19 Pandemic," *Atlanta Business Chronicle*, May 15, 2020. www.bizjournals.com.

Chapter Two: Keeping Society Safe and Functioning

12. Quoted in Brian Gingras, "The Rising Number of Deaths at Home Has NYPD Detectives Fighting an 'Invisible Bullet,'" CNN, April 10, 2020. www.cnn.com.
13. Quoted in Michael Daly, "What It's Like to Be a Paramedic in Brooklyn's Hot Zone," Daily Beast, March 27, 2020. www.thedailybeast.com.
14. Quoted in Heidi Groover, "What Does Safe Public Transit Look Like During COVID-19?," *Governing*, August 24, 2020. www.governing.com.
15. Quoted in Christina Capatides, "Truck Drivers, Grocery Store Workers and More Unsung Heroes of the Coronavirus Pandemic," CBS News, March 20, 2020. www.cbsnews.com.
16. Quoted in Sarah Scoles, "We're Not Heroes; We're Sacrificial.' Workers Carry the Burden of Colorado's Food Supply Chain," Colorado Public Radio, May 3, 2020. www.cpr.org.
17. Quoted in Melissa Chan, "'I've Never Been So Afraid.' 5 Employees on the Everyday Terror of Working in Grocery Stores During the Pandemic," *Time*, April 9, 2020. https://time.com.
18. Quoted in Chan, "'I've Never Been So Afraid.'"
19. Quoted in Nora Fleming, "Curbing Teacher Burnout During the Pandemic," Edutopia, May 8, 2020. www.edutopia.org.
20. Quoted in Alana Abramson, "The Country Won't Work Without Them. 12 Stories of People Putting Their Lives on the Line to Help Others During Coronavirus," *Time*, April 9, 2020. https://time.com.

Chapter Three: Turning the Tide

21. Quoted in Abby Visoulis, "From Homeless to Health Director: Meet the Woman Fighting to Flatten the Coronavirus Curve in Ohio," *Time*, April 9, 2020. https://time.com.
22. Quoted in Meredith Deliso, "'Unsafe': Women in Public Health Facing Pushback and Threats for Coronavirus Response," ABC News, July 3, 2020. https://abcnews.go.com.
23. Quoted in Lois R. Shea, "'Everyday Superheroes' Working to Help Homeless During Pandemic," New Hampshire Charitable Foundation, April 20, 2020. www.nhcf.org.
24. Quoted in Kevin Nathan, "Hartford Officer Continues Mission to Help the Homeless During a Pandemic," NBC Connecticut, May 14, 2020. www.nbcconnecticut.com.

25. Quoted in Grace Baek, "Navajo Nation Residents Face Coronavirus Without Running Water," WLNS, May 9, 2020. www.wlns.com.

26. Quoted in CNN, "With Navajo Nation Hit Hard by Covid-19, This CNN Hero's Mission to Help Vulnerable Elders Has a New Urgency," KVIA, July 30, 2020. https://kvia.com.

27. Quoted in Visiting Nurse Service of New York, "Partners in Care Home Health Aides: Providing Vital Care Through the Pandemic," 2020. www.vnsny.org.

28. Francis Collins, "Meet the Researcher Leading NIH's COVID-19 Vaccine Development Efforts," *NIH Director's Blog*, July 9, 2020. https://directorsblog.nih.gov.

29. Quoted in Karen Weintraub, "Why Volunteer for a Vaccine Clinical Trial? Duty, Love and a Willingness to Experiment, Participants Say," MSN, September 4, 2020. www.msn.com.

Chapter Four: Young Heroes

30. Quoted in Amanda Klarsfeld, "'This Will Pass': Teen Writes Letters to Help Others Feel Better During COVID-19," *South Florida Sun-Sentinel* (Fort Lauderdale, FL), August 6, 2020. www.sun-sentinel.com.

31. Quoted in Klarsfeld, "'This Will Pass.'"

32. Quoted in Aylin Salahifar, "Bay Area Teens Fight for Healthcare Heroes," Scot Scoop, May 4, 2020. https://scotscoop.com.

33. Quoted in Iris Samuels, "Tribes Turn to Musicians to Raise Kids' Awareness of COVID," *The Missoulian* (Missoula, MT), June 21, 2020. https://missoulian.com.

34. Quoted in Natalie Shepherd, "Milwaukee Teen, Crystal Russell, Works to Feed Those in Need," CBS58, July 22, 2020. www.cbs58.com.

35. Quoted in Jaime Dunaway, "How 2 Lakewood Teens Fed Thousands of Homeless During the Coronavirus Pandemic," *The Advocate*, August 5, 2020. https://lakewood.advocatemag.com.

36. Quoted in Bridget Shirvell, "Teens Are Helping Seniors Stay Connected During the Coronavirus Pandemic," *Teen Vogue*, April 1, 2020. www.teenvogue.com.

37. Quoted in Carrie Hodousek, "Difference Makers: South Bay Teens Create Friendship Network for Seniors," Radio.com, August 20, 2020. www.radio.com.

38. Quoted in Jennifer Maele, "Grocery Gatherers: Wayzata Teen Helps Out by Grocery Shopping for Those Most at Risk for COVID-19," CBS Minnesota, April 3, 2020. https://minnesota.cbslocal.com.

39. Quoted in Maele, "Grocery Gatherers."

Centers for Disease Control and Prevention (CDC)

www.cdc.gov/coronavirus/2019-ncov

The CDC is the nation's premier public health protection agency. The agency's website devotes significant space to coronavirus and COVID-19 facts and statistics. The site also has extensive information on who is at risk, protective measures, contact tracing, community response, schools and youth, and more.

Johns Hopkins Coronavirus Resource Center (CRC)

https://coronavirus.jhu.edu

The CRC, created and run by Johns Hopkins University & Medicine, is a continuously updated source of COVID-19 data and expert guidance. The center gathers and analyzes statistics and other information related to COVID-19 cases, testing, contact tracing, and vaccine research. The site also provides links to numerous articles from a variety of sources.

National Institute of Allergy and Infectious Diseases (NIAID)

www.niaid.nih.gov

The NIAID is one of the twenty-seven institutes and centers that make up the National Institutes of Health. Its website includes information about coronaviruses, the public health and government response to COVID-19, and treatment guidelines. It also provides details on volunteering for prevention clinical studies.

National Institutes of Health (NIH)

www.nih.gov/coronavirus

Part of the US Department of Health and Human Services, the NIH is the largest biomedical research agency in the world. Its website provides information on development of COVID-19 vaccines, testing, and treatments as well as links to other related topics.

US Food & Drug Administration (FDA)
www.fda.gov

The FDA regulates drugs, medical devices, and other products and oversees food safety. Its website provides pandemic-related statistics and information on protective equipment, treatments, and testing. It includes an extensive section of frequently asked questions about a variety of COVID-19 topics.

World Health Organization (WHO)
www.who.int/emergencies/diseases/novel-coronavirus-2019

Working within the framework of the United Nations, the WHO directs and coordinates global health issues. Its website features rolling coronavirus updates, situation reports, travel advice, facts about preventive measures such as masks, information on how the virus spreads, and more.

Additional resources: City, county, and state public health departments

Books

Emily Hudd, *Frontline Heroes*. North Mankato, MN: ABDO, 2020.

Douglas Hustad, *Understanding COVID-19*. North Mankato, MN: ABDO, 2020.

Hal Marcovitz, *The COVID-19 Pandemic: The World Turned Upside Down*. San Diego, CA: Reference Point Press, 2021.

Triumph Books, *American Heroes: Stories of Courage and Hope from the Front Lines of the Pandemic*. Chicago: Triumph, 2020.

Internet Sources

Boston, "Best of Boston 2020: The COVID-19 Heroes Edition," 2020. www.bostonmagazine.com.

Quentin Fottrell, "If Every American Started Wearing a Face Mask Today, This Is How Many Lives Could Be Saved," MarketWatch, August 10, 2020. www.marketwatch.com.

Good Teen News, "The Future Is in Good Hands," 2020. http://goodteennews.com.

Sandy Hingston, "Best of Philly: Here's to the Scientists and Frontline Heroes Fighting for Our Lives," *Philadelphia Magazine*, July 16, 2020. www.phillymag.com.

UAW, "Courage Against COVID-19: Members Face Down a Deadly Virus," June 29, 2020. https://uaw.org.

Randi Weingarten, "Heroes on the Frontlines of COVID-19," AFT, April 19, 2020. www.aft.org.

Note: Boldface page numbers indicate illustrations.